Reasons, Remedies And Treatments For Heartburns

Contents

Chapter 1 - What are the reasons for heartburns?

Excessive stomach acid leakage into the esophagus or lower throat is what leads to heartburns. Acid reflux which means acid flow back is a medical name used for stomach acid flow back from the stomach of the patient to the esophagus. Further acid reflux syndrome, heart reflux, acid burn and Gastrointestinal acid reflux disease are the terms which are used to explain the symptoms of heartburns. It is an ordeal which seriously disrupts the live of the sufferer especially who experience frequent symptoms of this distressing problem. The patient has to bear a constant uneasiness and pain while eating and drinking. Sleeping becomes difficult as the pain deepens when you lie down.

A majority of the people struggle with heartburns because of their eating habits, while very few suffer from this condition due to their genetic frame.

Heartburns take place when the lower esophageal sphincter between the stomach and the esophagus doesn't close up properly leading to severe damages to the esophagus. LES is extremely sensitive to a lot of foodstuffs which tend to make it wobbly. Some of the possible culprits that can cause heartburns include foods which are acidic such as oranges, spicy foods like enchiladas and sweet eatables like chocolates. Apart from these, there are various other factors which can develop gastroesophageal disorders. It has been revealed that consumption of alcohol or tobacco can cause the LES (Lower Esophageal Sphincter) not to close properly. Moreover, things like obesity, pregnancy etc. tend to put pressure or weight on stomach that causes the food consumed to flow back. Excessive amount of acid out of the stomach further triggers heartburn. Also, stress and tension are known to be the biggest causes of overstimulation of the gastric acid.

Thus, the patients undergoing this ordeal first need to make certain changes in their eating habits and lifestyles. Eating large portions of meals and that too full of fats and calories are the foremost things to say goodbye to. Lack of a good exercise routine and being always stressed out make your obese which directly affects you digestive system. The reasons of heartburns can cease if the patient stops smoking, eat small portions of meals at frequent intervals, avoids fatty and spicy foods, lose some weight and look for different ways to overcome stress. If the heartburns goes untreated, the condition can worsen leading to perilous diseases like ulcers, Barrett's esophagus, esophageal cancer etc. We shall discuss about all these aspects of this disease in the following chapters.

Chapter 2 - Types of heartburns

Heartburns are categorized under various types depending on factors like their cause, severity etc. Thus, before seeking a suitable treatment for this painful and distressing ordeal, it is good to know the type of heartburns you are undergoing. Some of the types of heartburns which are very common include-

Gastro Esophageal Reflux Disease-   Gastro

Esophageal Reflux Disease which is also known as Acid Reflux is the most serious and painful form of heartburns. GERD being a sign of a severe underlying problem is more than just a normal heartburn. If the patient suffers from heartburns more than one time in a week for many hours/days, there are more chances that he is suffering from Gastro Esophageal Reflux Disease and not just a simple heartburn. If not treated on time, it can even lead to many perilous health problems like halitosis, laryngitis, asthma, wheezing, interstitial fibrosis, gingivitis etc.

Pregnancy heartburns- Heartburn is one of the health problems which can be brought by pregnancy. However, the good part is that these heartburns go away after the infant is born. During pregnancy's third trimester, the pressure on the stomach increases which decelerate the digestive system and cause the acids to stay in stomach for long. This increases the chances of the digestive acids to flow back from the stomach to the esophagus giving rise to heartburns.

Chronic heartburns- Chronic heartburns are quite severe and occurs twice or thrice a week. Since such frequent attacks of heartburn can be a warning of more serious diseases like Gastro Esophageal Reflux Disease, it is advisable to get yourself examined by a specialized doctor to know the actual reason behind such recurrent heartburn attacks. Knowing the heartburn type you are suffering from make it quire easier to find out the causes for your heartburns.

Summer heartburns- Summer is a season for outings, enjoying the delicious cheese sandwiches and scrumptious fries and also for increased heartburns. The stifling high temperature combined with oily and fatty foodstuff leads to more chances of heartburn attacks. Thus, during summers it is advisable to stay away from acidic food and have light meals which are easy and quick to digest.

Nighttime heartburn- It is among the worst types of heartburns. While other heartburn attacks occur during daytime and thus it is easier to deal with them either by taking medicines or by resting, nighttime heartburn attacks the patient at night when their body is completely relaxed and not ready to handle such agonizing pain and uneasiness. However, there are still some ways to alleviate all these heartburns which shall be discussed in detailed in the next chapter.

Chapter 3 - Ways to alleviate heartburns

Heartburn is extremely painful and is an unpleasant burning sensation in the esophagus which happens due to excessive stomach acid. However, by taking certain steps you alleviate this distressing malady to a great extent. To overcome the ordeal of heartburn attacks, it is best to look for the causes first and then decide about the steps to be taken to assuage this problem. As mentioned earlier, heartburns occur when excessive stomach acid results in irritation in the esophagus. It happens if the lower esophageal sphincter is not sealed or closed properly. There are two chief reasons which results in such a state.

One major reason is overeating which fills up the stomach in excess. Thus, the obvious way to alleviate heartburn is to avoid eating too much even if your dining table is full of delicious oily and fatty foodstuff. Limiting yourself to only moderate meal portions can help you experience great results by getting you relieved from frequent heartburn attacks.

Another reason which leads to this problem is too much weight or pressure over the stomach. Such a condition is most common during pregnancy or obesity. Thus, for a pregnant lady a good posture, using a comfortable pillow, avoiding sleeping immediately after the meals etc. are some of the ways which highly reduces the discomfort. Ideally, it is best to go to bed 2-3 hours after eating. However, after pregnancy when the baby is born, all the symptoms of heartburns go away but in the case of obesity the only way to reduce the bouts of heartburns is to lose weight.

Some of the foodstuff which should be avoided by the patients of heartburns includes citrus fruits, chocolate, mustard, tomatoes, sodas, juice, coffee, vinegar etc. Foods with higher fat content lead to heartburns and thus fried and oily foodstuff should be avoided. Instead, incorporate certain alterations in your lifestyle to alleviate the pain and discomfort of heartburns. Follow a good exercise and diet regime including aloe Vera, chamomile tea, raw potatoes, marshmallows, turmeric etc.

Smoking is one of the major culprits of the painful heartburn bouts as it stimulates stomach acid production. Besides, stress also contributes to this agonizing condition. Thus along with following a good exercising and diet plan, quit smoking and stay away from stress. A few lifestyle modifications such as these can make a great difference in the life of a heartburn patient.

Chapter 4 - Dealing with persistent heartburns

Persistent heartburn being one of the worst forms of heartburns is extremely painful and attacks the patient twice or thrice a weak. Some of the symptoms of this ordeal include difficulty in swallowing, sore throat, coughing, chest pain with burning sensation and food getting back to the mouth even after swallowing. Seeking medical guidance is obviously the best way to go as remaining unchecked can lead to more severe complications. Acid flowing back to the esophagus can eventually result in serious damage. Constant heartburn if not treated on time could even result in diseases like ulcers in esophagus or stricture which implies the esophageal slims or narrows after a certain stage. The worst case may be Barrett's esophagus that in turn can result in esophageal cancer.

Fortunately, there are certain ways with the help of which the occurrence of heartburn symptoms can be highly reduced. The incidents of persistent heartburn attacks twice or thrice a week if remained unchecked can be undermining your healthiness. A specialist doctor can very well assess your present condition and opt for appropriate actions. Besides there are certain lifestyle alterations which can help you effectively deal with persistent heartburns.

To begin with, consider what you eat so that you can isolate the foodstuff that seems to correspond with a heartburn attack and eliminate that from your meal plan. Also watch out for the beverages you drink. For instance, if bouts of heartburns follow soon after consuming drinks like coffee, alcohol etc., cut them out of your diet or moderate. Besides, avoid eating fatty and oily foodstuff especially not within 3-4 hours of going to bed. Instead of large meals eat small frequent meals because when the stomach is too full, there is more likelihood of acid entering the esophagus.

Moreover, it is good to drink plenty of water if you are a heartburn patient as water is a healthy and natural neutralizer for acids. In addition, tight fitted clothes are also an unfavorable sign for heartburns. These are a few common lifestyle alterations regarding persistent heartburn. However, if the symptoms persist then it is advisable that you should see a doctor. Depending on your condition, they can give you the needed medicines and advice on how you can alleviate

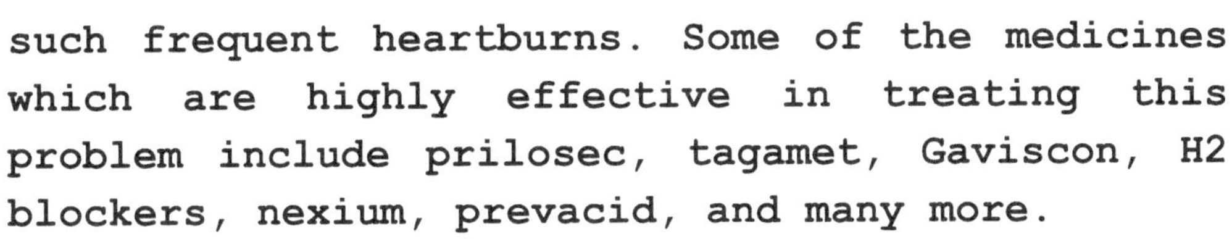
such frequent heartburns. Some of the medicines which are highly effective in treating this problem include prilosec, tagamet, Gaviscon, H2 blockers, nexium, prevacid, and many more.

Chapter 5 - Natural treatments for heartburns

Heartburn is a medical condition associated with digestive system where the stomach acid flow back to the esophagus and cause burning sensations under the sternum and breastbone. It varies from mild and sporadic to serious and chronic. They are classified into various forms depending on their severity. For instance, chronic heartburns may be a sign of some serious problems like gastritis, hiatal hernia, peptic ulcer etc. Fortunately, there are copious treatments available for heartburns. They can be dealt with antacids like Mylant, Riopan, Maalax etc. However, these can only lessen the pain temporarily and do not provide a lasting healing effect.

One of the most imperative and effective steps to treat this problem is to make some serious alterations in your lifestyles. Some of the things to be avoided in case you want to get relieved form the painful symptoms of this disease are alcohol, cigarettes, fatty food, spicy food, junk food etc. Quitting all these would lower down the level of acid in your body providing better functioning of the organs. Also, avoid sleeping immediately after your meals.

Ideally, one should go to bed three to four hours after eating. It is also advisable to take smaller meals at frequent time intervals instead of taking three big meals as smaller meals give sufficient time to your system for digesting the food.

In addition, going for regular walks too helps in alleviating the discomfort caused due to this ordeal. Besides, as ginger is good to treat this condition, you can take it as ginger tablets, ginger tea and even in its raw form. Apart from this, aloe Vera juice, chamomile, fennel tea etc. also help in curing heartburn. There are some methods to speed up the digestive process as well such as taking cumin seeds along with a glass of water or an apple after consuming your meals. It is also advisable to drink plenty of water. Water if consumed in a good amount as per your body needs can charge up the rate of metabolism and purifies your body system which ultimately helps in improving digestion.

Light exercises can also help in relieving diseases associated with the digestion system. Devoting just a few minutes to moderate physical activities in a day such as stretching, walking, jogging etc. would improve your circulation as well as digestive muscle movements and thereby helps in digesting food easily. All the mentioned natural treatments would help to alleviate burning, choking and chest pain caused due to heartburn. Plus, you would feel better both physically as well as mentally.

Chapter 6 - Some effective home Remedies for heartburns

Presently, home remedies to treat heartburn is the most preferred way to purely heal the heartburn disorders along with improving overall physical health. Even the medical professionals are realizing the effectiveness of various home treatments. The discomfort caused by heartburn attacks is usually described as a deep and painful burning sensation arising from the stomach to the middle of the chest. In severe cases, it also results in injuries in the esophagus. Fortunately, just by opting for a few changes in your diet plan, it is possible to get rid of the heartburn disease. To begin with, trim down the number of meals you take in a day to smaller meal portions so that the food gets enough time to digest.

Natural heartburn cures can be found in many everyday meals, drinks and herbs. You can begin with your natural reflux remedy by simply including some indigestion foods in your diet which are soft as well as moist to be digested quickly. Soft foodstuff can easily flow to your stomach allowing your esophagus or sphincter to initiate healing. Keeping away from hard and crunchy foods is paramount for the heartburn patients as they may worsen the problem. The simplest remedy is to drink plenty of water as it keeps your LES (Lower Esophageal Sphincter) muscle flap firmly closed over your stomach. Such a tight seal would not let the stomach acid to flow into the esophagus. Water also allows quick reproduction of the tissue cells.

Honey is also a terrific heartburn natural home remedy. Since, this problem of heartburns is caused due to damaging of the tissues in esophagus and sphincter, having three to four spoons of honey every day can help in repairing these tissues. Another ingredient which is awful in taste but good to cure heartburn is apple cider vinegar. To make it taste better you can add in it some water and honey. It has been proven that taking one spoon of this mix daily can highly improve your acid levels and food digestion.

For instant relief, you can have a solution of coriander juice, one tablespoon of cumin seeds, one glass of water and a pinch of salt. Taking carrot juice, coconut water and chewing basil leaves also helps in get rid of heartburn. If you do not wish to go for the high-priced medical prescriptions which can result in many side-effects and only treat the heartburn symptoms and not its reasons, then without a doubt you would genuinely like to consider the above mentioned extremely useful home remedies.

Chapter 7 - How to deal with heartburns during pregnancy?

Many women suffer from heartburns during the third trimester of their pregnancy. As the baby grows, he/she begins to put pressure or weight on the stomach which ultimately results the stomach acid to flow in the esophagus. It causes a burning sensation under the sternum and breastbone known as heartburns. Although heartburns during pregnancy have no side effects on the baby and the symptoms also vanish as soon as the infant is born, however before that the suffering can be pretty uncomfortable. If you are also one of the ladies experiencing the incidence of heartburns during pregnancy, here are some tips which you can follow to get relief.

- As this problem is directly associated with your digestive system, special attention should be given to what you eat, when you eat and in what quality you eat. Take small and frequent portions of meals and slowly chew whatever you eat.

- Avoid foods that can trigger or activate gastrointestinal distress such as alcoholic beverages, caffeine beverages, chocolates, spicy foods, acidic foodstuff(like tomatoes, mustard, citrus fruits, vinegar), mint products, fatty or oily foods, processed meats(bologna, bacon, hot dogs, sausage) and highly seasoned foods.

* Avoid drinking too much water during meals. This causes stomach distension which can further trigger heartburn.

* Quit smoking if you do as it is one of those habits which may lead to many serious diseases including heartburns.

* Avoid wearing such clothes which emphasis your tummy or waist as it can result in heartburns. Instead wear loose and comfortable clothing.

* Avoid lying down or sleeping immediately after your meals. The best is to go to bed after three to four hours after eating food. This gives sufficient time to your body for digesting the food.

* Sleep over extra pillows which would slightly elevate the upper body and thereby ward off the stomach acid to rise up in the chest.

* Also a good posture can reduce your discomfort to a great extent. So, be sure you

stand straight as well as sit straight. Bending on the knees instead of the waist would reduce pressure on your ever-growing tummy.

- Taking herbal tea such as slippery elm, spearmint, chamomile and ginger tea. These would help in providing relief from heartburn during pregnancy.

By following all the above stated tips and suggestions; you can enjoy a relaxed and comfortable pregnancy without facing any incidence of discomforting bouts of heartburn.

Chapter 8 - Connection between Heartburns and arthritis

If the heartburn symptoms occur more than thrice a week for a persistent period of two to three weeks, then in that case the symptoms are deemed chronic. If one is suffering from incessant heartburn, it is quite essential to find out if there has been any modification in diet, increased stress, and increased consumption of alcohol or the intake of strong medicine for a prolonged period. For a confirmed chronic heartburn there must have occurred a substantial change if the diet of an individual and other aspects of his lifestyle have not altered or changed in that case it is probably an indication of some other medical problem. In this case, it is very essential that one should be aware of the reasons and circumstances as an individual using natural remedies or self-treatment in order to fight against the chronic heartburn is probably covering the symptoms of some more serious problem.

Usually, heartburn is caused by the flow of acid and contents into the esophagus from the stomach and thereby causing the acid to irritate the sensitive lining of the stomach. Quite often, when an individual suffers from chronic heartburn, he is having an inconsistent dietary habits or he is having foods or drinks which is quite high in its acidic content and thus the digestive system functions and eventually produces excessive acids. In such cases a counter medication will combat the burning sensation which will disappear as soon as the substance is processed. However if the symptoms are persistent over a period of time, the chronic heartburn is probably diagnosed and would be treated with appropriate and prescription medications.

Also, heartburn can be a possible symptom of medical conditions like GERD or gastroesophageal reflux disease, hiatal hernia, pregnancy, peptic ulcer, acid regurgitation, stomach related disorders and even coughing for a prolonged period. The medications for the treatment of heart problems, respiratory problems, arthritis, blood pressure, osteoporosis, insomnia, depression, anxiety, cancer and Parkinson's disease are even known to be the cause of heartburn.

The commonly used drugs to treat arthritis earlier are NSAIDS or the non-steroidal anti-inflammatory drugs. Though the reflux symptoms or the heartburn symptoms are quite common with the use of non-steroidal anti-inflammatory medications, these symptoms correlate very badly with bleeding from the tract of gastro intestine. The gastrointestinal symptoms such as bloating or abdominal pain or heartburn are commonly found in the patients who are using the NSAIDS. This as a result increases difficulty in treating arthritis and also the adverse effects which are related to the arthritis treatment. Also, it is very difficult to predict the duration of time an arthritis patient is supposed to be treated with NSAIDS.

Chapter 9 – Heartburns - should be taken seriously or not?

Majority of people do not take the problem of heartburn seriously till it turns into a chronic condition. The result being pretty obvious is worse than expected. There are scores of reasons why heartburns should be taken seriously. In the initial stages, heartburn can be easily remedied. All you need to do is to take an antacid to get back to normal. But when the problem aggravates you have to go for those super-sized bottles of antacid tablets. Though these multiple flavored sugary pills provide fast relief but sadly just on a temporary basis.

And then you start realizing that you require something else probably more effective and thus go for some other over-the-counter product offering 12-24 hours relief. For months or possibly years you rely on these over-the counter remedies to keep the bouts of heartburn under control. However, when something goes wrong in your body which needs medical attention and you realize that now your heartburn problem has become an intimidating malady with intensifying pain resulting in sleepless nights, do you really think it is the right time to visit a doctor? If not, heartburn should be taken seriously from the very beginning when you experience your first ever heartburn attack in life.

The doctor hands you a big list of what foods and beverages to avoid, tells you to drop weight and along with that gives you a medical prescription to go for. However, it becomes difficult to follow such a restricted routine when you know that you have never ever bothered about what you eat and how much you eat. If you do not want something like this to happen to you as well, it is advisable to see a specialist doctor when you experience the symptoms of heartburn for the very first time.

This disease if not taken seriously can lead to some perilous diseases such as cancer, ulcer, hiatal hernia, Barrett's esophagus and many more. So, remember no medications or pills would work once you reach an incurable stage of heartburn. Thus, make some positive lifestyle alterations so as to keep your digestive procedure in a good working condition such as quit smoking, follow an exercise routine, avoid lying down immediately after meals, avoid consuming alcoholic beverages, tobacco, oily foods, spicy foods, acidic foods, fatty foods, junk food, citric fruits, chocolate, caffeine, peppermint etc. All these things would keep you healthy both physically as well as mentally.

Chapter 10 - Right diet to alleviate heartburns

If you are suffering from heartburn or the Gastroesophageal Reflux Disease (GERD) you can probably get rid of the symptoms by merely changing or altering your lifestyle. Using the prescription drugs might be a final resource if one tries using these small changes before. There are diets which can effectively reduce the heartburn to a considerable level. Your dietary habits play a very important role in treating this problem and controlling it.

As many individuals have heartburn flare ups late in the evening. So, in this case it is advisable to put a curb on your nighttime eating. Try to have your meal 2-3 hours before you go to sleep. If you actually want to get rid of the heartburn symptoms, you should be aware of the fact that the diet you have and the foods you consume can be a major source of this digestive disorder. Foods with high acidic content are more likely to cause acid reflux and you should avoid few drinks like caffeinated beverages, juice and alcohol to get rid of the heartburn symptoms.

Also, foods which have high fat like chocolates, hot foods having peppers are likely to cause the problem of heartburn. . If the foods that you consume are high in fat and acidic content like citrus fruits and tomatoes, you should reduce the intake of such foods and try to include more safe and healthy foods which will considerably reduce the frequency of heartburn. The foods which are low in fat and acidic content are safer like bananas, pears and apples are better choices as compared to oranges. Also, grilled, boiled or baked skinless, chicken and baked, broiled or boiled seafood are better than the fried chicken and hamburgers.

The most recommended ways in order to considerably reduce the frequency of heartburn include the dietary changes along with the lifestyle changes. For instance it is better to have small and light meals every few hours rather than having a large meal once or twice a day. Also, if an individual is overweight, having more frequent smaller meals may help to lose weight by increasing the metabolism rate and maintaining proper levels of blood glucose.

Also, if you are having junk foods at all times then it is the time to stop the consumption of junk food which is more likely to cause frequent heartburn attacks. It is very important to include fresh fruits and vegetables in your diet. By making simple changes in your eating habits and diet plan you can significantly improve your digestion and health and this will eventually decrease your susceptibility to heartburn.

Conclusion

Excessive stomach acid leakage into the esophagus or lower throat is what leads to heartburns. Acid reflux which means acid flow back is a medical term used for stomach acid flow back from the stomach of the patient to the esophagus. It is a digestive disorder which seriously disrupts the life of the sufferer particularly the one who is experiencing frequent symptoms of this distressing problem.

Heartburn is actually a burning pain which starts from the back of breastbone and ribs and then radiates upwards to the throat. It is caused by the acid flowing into the esophagus from the stomach. Due to the corrosive nature of the acid, it irritates and inflames the esophagus and causes the problem of heartburn. Also, it varies from mild and sporadic to serious and chronic. Thus if you are suffering from this digestive disorder you should consult a doctor. Also by implementing few changes in your dietary habits and lifestyle you can get rid of the symptoms of heartburn. if in case the heartburn symptoms occur more than thrice a week for a persistent period of two to three weeks, then in that case the symptoms are deemed chronic and you should consult a doctor before going for any self-treatment.

Articles

Here are some short articles given as "food-for-thought".

Cure heartburn by avoiding these food items

Most commonly the problem of heartburn is caused by the kind of foods that we eat. Having unhealthy and fatty foods can increase the production of acid in your stomach. It also slows down the digestion process which in turn causes heartburn. People who suffer from acid reflux or heartburn should try to find out that which food items can increase this problem so that they can avoid any such food. To make it easier for you, here is a list of some food items which can generally cause heartburn:

- Fruits: Citrus fruits, such as orange, lemon can cause the production of acid. Other than these, the juices of grapefruit and cranberry can also increase the problem of heartburn.
- Vegetables: tomato is one vegetable which is very acidic in nature. Other vegetables such as raw onion, pepper and chilies should also be avoided.
- Dairy products: Any type of dairy items, such as milk shake, sour cream, ice cream, eggs, cheese also increases the chances of heartburn.
- Meats: meats are very high in fat content and take a lot of time to digest. Try to avoid meats like beef, Buffalo wings, chicken nuggets etc.
- Greasy foods: Foods which are fried are not good for your digestive system. It is better to avoid cheeseburgers, French fries and other fast foods which are fried.
- Beverages: Excessive intake of alcohol, soda and other beverages which contain caffeine, like tea and coffee are the major causes of heartburn.
- Chocolate: consuming chocolate in any form, be it eating or drinking, is best avoided if you are suffering from heartburn.

The best way to avoid this problem is to avoid any such food which is high in sugar, fat, spices or caffeine. All these items are known causes of heartburn. Try to eat slowly and have smaller portions to avoid hampering your digestion system.

Determine the heartburn type to find out the best remedy

Heartburn is very common digestive problem. Before one looks for a solution for heartburn, it is advisable to first understand the type of heartburn a person is suffering from. One might found it surprising but the fact is that the heartburns are categorized into different types and these types depend upon the cause and the severity of the problem.

One of the most common types of heartburn is the summer heartburn. The stifling heat when combined with fatty foods is likely to make a person more vulnerable to heartburns. If you experience heartburn in this way then you are most likely to suffer from summer heartburn. In this case it is advisable to have light meals which can be easily digested and avoid the acidic foods. Another common type of heartburn is the pregnancy heartburn. During the pregnancy the pressure against the stomach increases which tends to slow down the digestion and because of this the digestive acids remain in your stomach for an extended period. This eventually increases the possibility of acid flow back into the esophagus from the stomach and results in heartburn.

The nighttime heartburn is another type of heartburn which is the most painful and the worst form. The nighttime heartburn usually occurs because of the reason that our body lies in the same position for many hours which tends to relax the esophageal sphincter and the flow of acid into the esophagus becomes easier.

Another common type of the heartburn is the chronic heartburn which is a term used for heartburn attacks which occur twice or thrice a week and is generally more severe. It is advisable to consult a doctor before finding a remedy to treat the chronic heartburn. Knowing and understanding the type of heartburn, one is suffering from makes it easier for him to know the cause and finding the suitable remedy to treat the problem.

Home remedies – finding natural cure for heartburn

Many people suffer from the problem of heartburn in their daily life. This problem is becoming more common each day. The biggest contributors to this problem are our unhealthy lifestyle habits and the kind of food that we take. Eating food that is high in fat, affects our digestive system. It increases the production of acid in the stomach, which in turn causes heartburn. This problem can be avoided by changing our lifestyle and by including healthy food items in our diet. In case you are suffering from the problem of heartburn, then you can try the following home remedies:

- Baking soda: Baking soda is considered very effective to cure heartburn as the bicarbonate in it helps to neutralize the acid in the stomach. Take a glass of warm water and mix a tablespoon of baking soda in it. It should be taken immediately when the symptoms appear.
- Banana: Banana is good for your system. People who regularly suffer from the problem of heartburn should make it a habit to eat a banana daily.

- Apple: Another fruit which can be beneficial for you is the apple. You can have some slices after taking your meal.
- Gum: You can chew a gum after your meal. It helps in digestion of the food and will help to avoid heartburn.
- Honey: Honey is also proven to be beneficial for you because of its antioxidant property. You can take about two spoonful of honey after your meal.
- Garlic: Raw garlic is famous for its antibiotic properties. Chewing a clove, immediately when the symptoms of heartburn appear, will help to relieve the problem.
- Water: Drinking adequate amount of water daily detoxifies your body by diluting stomach acids and will also keep you well hydrated.

Obesity is also a major cause of heartburn. Regular exercise or any other physical activity helps you to maintain your weight and can also improve your digestive system.

Identifying the symptoms of heartburn

The acid reflux, more commonly known as heartburn, is experienced by a large number of order to prevent heartburn, it is _ for you to understand that what a _ly is heartburn and what are its symptoms. Heartburn is the condition when you feel a burning sensation in your stomach. It generally occurs when the acid in your stomach, flows into the esophagus, instead of getting digested. It causes a burning feeling in the throat and chest. It is better to properly identify the symptoms of heartburn before starting any remedies or medication. Here is a list of some common symptoms that a person may feel during heartburn:

- Burning sensation: the burning sensation does not actually occur in the heart or the stomach but can be felt near the breastbone. That is why most people complain of a burning sensation in the chest area during heartburn.
- Sore throat: the next part that gets affected the most, after the chest, is the throat. You might feel an unusual soreness in your throat, especially in the back area, which is very similar to the feeling of burning.
- Bitter taste: when a person is suffering from heartburn he will usually feel a bitter taste in his mouth. This bitter or sour taste in the mouth or throat is actually caused by the acid.

- Difficulty in swallowing: Having such soreness in your throat makes it difficult to swallow anything. You can feel as if you have a lump in your throat which is making it hard for you to swallow.
- Coughing: though generally it is not associated with heartburn but cough can also occur. As the top portion of your lungs gets affected, it can cause cough very similar to asthma.

The most prominent symptom of heartburn is that this condition occurs mainly after eating spicy or fried foods. This problem can be easily avoided by improving your eating habits.

Improve your lifestyle and get rid of heartburn symptoms

Heartburn is a common digestive disorder and is inflicting more and more individuals today. When it comes to the treatment of this common problem it is very essential to find out the origin or the root cause of the problem. The biggest reason for the individuals suffering from this problem is their lifestyle. Today, the individuals are leading a very unhealthy lifestyle which is the major reason why they are inflicted with various types of ailments.

In order to get rid of the symptoms of heartburn you need to improve your lifestyle to increase your overall productivity in the daily chores. The individuals suffering from heartburn need to check out their dietary habits. If you are having junk food at all times then it is the time to stop the consumption of junk food which is likely to cause frequent heartburn attacks. It is very important to include fresh fruits and vegetables in your diet to get rid of the heartburn symptoms. By making simple changes in your eating habits and diet plan you can significantly improve your digestion and health and this will eventually decrease your susceptibility to heartburn.

Another very important factor which influences the susceptibility to heartburn and many other ailments is sleep. Having adequate amount of sleep is very important in order to have a healthy living. During sleep your body undergoes the process of healing and regeneration. So, if you are not getting good amount of sleep for a prolonged period you are more likely to suffer from the consequences and heartburn is one of them. Stress is another very important factor which causes many conditions and diseases. Too much stress is not good for health and you should find out the ways to de-stress and relax yourself in order to have a healthy lifestyle. By implementing these small changes you can improve your health and get rid of the symptoms of heartburn.

Natural remedies- an effective treatment for heartburn

Heartburn, a digestive ailment is a very common medical condition today. The common symptoms are sore throat, sensation in the chest, bitter taste of mouth, difficulty in swallowing and coughing. These are the few symptoms of this digestive problem and one can treat it by taking a suitable medication. Today, thousands of individuals are suffering from this digestive ailment with different levels and frequencies.

In order to effectively deal with this problem, one needs to follow a lifestyle and a balanced diet which can successfully help to get rid of the symptoms. You can considerably reduce the occurrence of heartburn attacks if you follow certain tips which will help you to increase the productivity in your daily chores. To get rid of this digestive problem you should avoid the intake of acidic and spicy foods. The foods like oranges, tomatoes, grapefruit, chilies, pepper and vinegar are likely to cause frequent heartburn attacks in the individuals.

Also, it is advisable to those suffering from heartburn to have fat free foods and avoid oily foods as they can cause more severe heartburns in some individuals. Also, you should have light meals during the day instead of having one heavy meal. Heavy meals are likely to cause acid reflux problem. So, it is advisable to take short breaks between the meals and have light meals. Further, you should avoid the intake of carbonated drinks and the drinks having caffeine. A healthy alternative for these is to have ginger tea or yogurt. One of the most effective drinks to get rid of this problem is the lemon water which can reduce the severity of a problem to a considerable level. Also, it is advisable to avoid having snacks before going to sleep. By using these helpful tips you can get rid of this digestive problem and can improve your lifestyle.

Tips to avoid heartburn at night

A large number of people complain about heartburn during the night. Heartburn occurring at night is considered worse that the day because of many factors. First of all it disturbs your sleep and can disrupt your sleep pattern by keeping you awake. Another factor is that waking up to a burning sensation in your chest and throat can make you very uneasy at night. So the next morning you will wake up looking fatigued and worn out. By practicing the following remedies you can avoid this problem:

- Avoid heavy meal: Our food gets digested more easily during the day as compared to the night. Try to have a light meal at night and avoid eating food that is fried or too spicy as it produces more acid.
- Do not smoke or drink: You should not smoke or drink alcohol late in the night as it can relax the LES, which can cause the burning sensation of heartburn.
- Sit straight: Your sitting posture is very important as it affects your digestive system. Always eat on the table and sit straight with your back against the chair.

- Do not lie down immediately: You should never lie down immediately after having your dinner. At least give a gap of two to three hours, between your dinner and sleeping time.

- Drink water: Drinking water before taking your meal will help you to feel full and can avoid overeating. Also you should not drink too much water during the meal.

- Elevate head of the bed: Raise the head of your bed by about four to six inches. It will prevent the acid from flowing back into esophagus.

- Do not exercise: Never exercise or indulge in some heavy physical activity right after your meal. You should give some time for the food to get digested.

Also avoid tight clothes. Do not wear very tight clothes in the night to avoid putting any pressure on your stomach. You will sleep much better in loose and comfortable clothes.

Treatment for heartburn

Heartburn is a very common digestive ailment. One can choose an appropriate medicine or treatment and can also find a suitable natural remedy for its treatment. Depending upon the frequency of attacks and the symptoms it is advisable to consult a doctor. Also, one can use the herbal remedy or an antacid product to treat the occasional heartburn. Heartburn is caused by an excessive flow of acid into the esophagus from the stomach. An effective medicine for heartburn treatment helps to neutralize the acid and relieves the sign and symptoms. The individuals having frequent heartburn attacks need to check out their lifestyle and dietary changes.

One of the effective ways to significantly reduce the occurrence of heartburn attacks is to reduce the intake of acidic foods in your diet. The foods like citrus fruits, tomatoes, fried foods and chocolates are responsible for the occurrence of frequent attacks. Before going for a treatment to cure the chronic heartburn, you need to check out your dietary habits and also try to know about the foods which cause sensitivity particularly if you are having occasional heartburn attacks.

Another effective way to cure this problem is to improve your dietary habits as the individuals who suffer from the chronic heartburn need to have light and small meals after regular intervals rather than having a large meal 1- 2 times a day. Overweight individuals are probably more vulnerable to frequent heartburn attacks so, an efficient and helpful heartburn treatment plan should include changing your diet and also the frequency of your meals. Besides, the kind of drinks you have can also be one of the reasons for frequent occurrence of heartburns. Coffee, alcohol, regular sodas, fruit juices and diet sodas can cause the occurrence of heartburn in some individuals. An efficient treatment program will help you to identify the changes that you need to make out in your diet and lifestyle and helps you to cure the problem.

Understanding the causes of heartburn

The burning sensation that you feel after eating a heavy meal is known as heartburn. It is commonly experienced by a large number of people all over the world. The main reasons for the occurrence of heartburn are associated with your food intake and lifestyle habits. By understanding the causes of heartburn it becomes easy to avoid this problem. Here is a list of some factors which can contribute in causing the heartburn:

- Spice and fried food: Having unhealthy and fatty foods is the biggest reason behind the occurrence of heartburn. The fried and spicy foods contain a high amount of fat and are not easily digested by our body.

- Heavy meal at dinner: Eating a heavy meal in the dinner increases the pressure in your stomach. Also people who eat very fast also tend to suffer from heartburn more than others.

- Lying down after a meal: Your stomach takes time to digest the food. Lying down just after having a meal causes the acid to flow from the stomach to the esophagus, which in turn causes the heartburn.

- Smoking and alcohol: The bad habits of excessive smoking and alcohol consumption are the major reasons for heartburn. Smoking and alcohol intake relaxes the esophageal sphincter that allows the acid to enter the stomach and causes heartburn.

- Indigestion: Other unhealthy habits related to food, such as eating heavy meals, not chewing your food properly, having foods which are full of fat and spices, affect your digestion system. It also increases the production of acid in your stomach which then gives rise to the problem of heartburn.

- Caffeine: Frequent and large intake of caffeine induced beverages like coffee, tea and soda also causes the acid to enter the esophagus.

You should try to analyze that what causes heartburn in your case because only after identifying the right cause, you can get rid of this problem.

What you can do to avoid heartburn?

Our unhealthy eating and lifestyle habits are the main causes of the problem of heartburn or acid reflex. It is generally caused by the acid in our stomach. When this acid enters the esophagus, it causes a burning sensation in throat and chest. This problem can cause a lot of inconvenience and pain. By keeping a check on what we eat and how we eat our food, we can avoid this problem. Below mentioned are some healthy habits that you should incorporate in your lifestyle:

- Eat healthy food: Make healthy foods a part of your diet. Avoid having foods which have high amount of fat or spices. Your method of cooking should also be healthy; it means that you should avoid frying your food in butter or oil.

- Eat yoghurt: A major cause of heartburn is indigestion. Yoghurt contains a lot of good bacteria which help to make your digestion system strong and also improve your immunity.
- Drink water: Water detoxifies your system from all unwanted components. It will help to keep your body well hydrated, so that you can avoid other unhealthy beverages, such as tea, coffee etc.
- Eat smaller portions: heartburn generally occurs when you put pressure on your stomach. In order to avoid that you should eat smaller portions of food at regular intervals, rather than having three big meals a day.
- Eat slowly: Take time to chew your food properly so that it can be digested easily. Eating your food slowly will help you to feel full and can thus avoid overeating.
- Watch your weight: heartburn is also linked to obesity. Keep a check on your food intake and your weight. Include exercises and other physical activities in your routine.

The problem of heartburn is mainly caused by unhealthy eating and lifestyle habits. By changing your lifestyle you can easily avoid this problem.

About the Author

C.X. Cruz was born in Puerto Rico and have lived in the New York City area since he was 14 years old. He holds graduate degrees from the State University of New York and Honolulu University in Computer Science. He has worked for European investment banks such as UBS, and for American banks such as Goldman Sachs. His hobbies include forestry and rowing.

As a very young graduate student, Cruz thought of publishing books. It was extremely difficult to publish a book using the traditional methods 30 years ago. He gave up on this publishing dream back then. Thankfully, there are numerous ways to become a self-publisher today. The internet has democratized many businesses such book publishing. Cruz can bring you great content and a great price. Never stop reading and learning. Cruz knows you will enjoy reading his books!

Legal

Use of this product indicates your acceptance of the "No Liability" policy. If you do not agree with our "No Liability" policy, then you are not permitted to use or distribute this product (if applicable.) Failure to read this notice in its entirety does not void your agreement to this policy should you decide to use this product.

Applicable law may not allow the limitation or exclusion of liability or incidental or consequential damages, so the above limitation or exclusion may not apply to you. The liability for damages, regardless of the form of the action, shall not exceed the actual fee paid for the product.

InDigitalWorks.com

Copyright